Workbook

For

30 Days 2 Shredz

Reprogram Your Mind and Metabolism to Torch Fat, Sculpt Muscle and Create Your Dream Body in 30 Days or Less

Alex Willowbrooks

Copyright

No part of this book may be reproduced in any written, electronic, recording, or photocopying without written permission of the publisher or author.

The exception would be in the case of brief quotations embodied in the critical articles or reviews and pages where permission is specifically granted by the publisher or author.

Although every precaution has been taken to verify the accuracy of the information contained herein, the author and publisher assume no responsibility for any errors or omissions. No liability is assumed for damages that may result from the use of the information contained within.

All Right Reserved@2023 Alex Willowbrooks

Disclaimer

This Workbook is an Unofficial Companion to the original book. It is not endorsed, sponsored, or associated with the original author or publisher of the original book.

All Views and opinions expressed in this workbook are those of "Alex Willowbrooks" and do not necessarily reflect the views and opinions of the author or publisher of the original book.

Alex Willowbrooks

This Workbook Belongs To:

_____

CONTENTS

HOW TO USE THIS WORKBOOK

This workbook is a companion guide to the book "30 Days 2 Shredz". It is designed to help you reach your weight loss goals by providing you with detailed chapter by chapter summaries, key points of each chapter, interactive exercise questions, and goals and actionable plans.

How to Use This Workbook

Read the chapter summaries: The chapter summaries provide a quick overview of the key points of each chapter. This will help you to get a sense of what each chapter covers and to identify the information that is most relevant to you.

Study the key points: The key points of each chapter provide a more detailed overview of the important information in that chapter. This is where you will find the most actionable advice for reaching your weight loss goals.

Complete the interactive exercise questions: The interactive exercise questions will help you to apply the information from the book to your own life. This is where you will develop your own goals and actionable plans for weight loss.

Set goals and create actionable plans: The goals and actionable plans section will help you to put everything you have learned into action. This is where you will create a plan that is specific, measurable, achievable, relevant, and time-bound.

Conclusion

This workbook is a valuable resource for anyone who is serious about reaching their weight loss goals. By following the steps outlined in this guide, you will be well on your way to success.

Here are some additional tips for using this workbook:

Use the workbook alongside the book: The workbook is designed to be used alongside the book. This will help you to get the most out of both resources.

Take your time: Don't try to rush through this workbook. Take your time to read the chapter summaries, study the key points, and complete the interactive exercise questions.

Be honest with yourself: When you are setting goals and creating actionable plans, be honest with yourself about your strengths and weaknesses. This will help you to create a plan that is realistic and achievable.

Get support: Don't be afraid to get support from friends, family, or a weight loss coach. Having people to support you can make a big difference in your success.

I hope this guide has persuaded you to use this workbook to reach your weight loss goals. With hard work and dedication, you can achieve anything you set your mind to.

INTRODUCTION

The introduction of the book begins by discussing the importance of having a positive mindset when it comes to achieving your fitness goals. The authors argue that if you believe you can achieve your goals, you are more likely to succeed. They also discuss the importance of setting realistic goals and making gradual changes to your lifestyle.

The introduction then goes on to provide an overview of the 30-day program. The program is divided into three phases: detox, shredding, and maintenance. The detox phase is designed to cleanse the body of toxins and prepare it for weight loss. The shredding phase is the main part of the program and involves following a strict diet and exercise regimen. The maintenance phase is designed to help readers keep the weight off after they have completed the program.

The introduction also discusses the importance of supplements in supporting weight loss and muscle building. The authors recommend a variety of supplements, including protein powder, creatine, and fish oil.

Finally, the introduction provides a few words of encouragement to readers. The authors remind readers that they are not alone and that they can achieve their goals with hard work and dedication.

Here are some additional thoughts on the introduction of the book:

The authors do a good job of explaining the importance of mindset and how it can affect your results.

The program is well-structured and easy to follow.

The book provides motivation and support throughout the program.

Overall, the introduction of the book is positive and inspiring. It sets the tone for the rest of the book and makes readers feel like they can achieve their goals.

CHAPTER ONE
The Mindset of a Shred

Chapter 1 discusses the importance of mindset when it comes to achieving your fitness goals. The authors argue that if you believe you can achieve your goals, you are more likely to succeed. They also discuss the importance of setting realistic goals and making gradual changes to your lifestyle.

The authors begin by discussing the difference between a "dreamer" and a "doer." Dreamers are people who have goals but never take action to achieve them. Doers are people who take action, even when it is difficult. The authors argue that if you want to achieve your fitness goals, you need to be a doer.

The authors then discuss the importance of setting realistic goals. They argue that if you set goals that are too difficult, you are more likely to give up. They recommend setting goals that are challenging but achievable.

The authors also discuss the importance of making gradual changes to your lifestyle. They argue that if you try to change too much too quickly, you are more likely to fail. They recommend making small changes that you can stick with over time.

The authors provide several examples of how to change your mindset to achieve your fitness goals. For example, they recommend telling yourself positive affirmations every day. They also recommend surrounding yourself with positive people who support your goals.

The authors conclude the chapter by reminding readers that they are not alone. They are all on a journey to achieve their fitness goals. They encourage readers to never give up on their dreams.

Here are some additional thoughts on Chapter 1:

The authors do a good job of explaining the importance of mindset and how it can affect your results.

The examples that the authors provide are helpful and inspiring.

The chapter is well-written and easy to follow.

Key Points of Chapter 1

The importance of mindset: The authors argue that your mindset is the most important factor in determining whether or not you will achieve your fitness goals. If you believe you can achieve your goals, you are more likely to succeed.

The difference between dreamers and doers: Dreamers are people who have goals but never take action to achieve them. Doers are people who take action, even when it is difficult. The authors argue that if you want to achieve your fitness goals, you need to be a doer.

The importance of setting realistic goals: The authors argue that if you set goals that are too difficult, you are more likely to give up. They recommend setting goals that are challenging but achievable.

The importance of making gradual changes to your lifestyle: The authors argue that if you try to change too much too quickly, you are more likely to fail. They recommend making small changes that you can stick with over time.

How to change your mindset: The authors provide several examples of how to change your mindset to achieve your fitness goals. For example, they recommend telling yourself positive affirmations every day. They also recommend surrounding yourself with positive people who support your goals.

Never give up: The authors conclude the chapter by reminding readers that they are not alone. They are all on a journey to achieve their fitness goals. They encourage readers to never give up on their dreams.

Here are some additional thoughts on the key points of Chapter 1:

The authors do a good job of explaining the importance of mindset and how it can affect your results.

The examples that the authors provide are helpful and inspiring.

The chapter is well-written and easy to follow.

Overall, Chapter 1 is an important chapter in the book. It provides readers with the tools they need to change their mindset and achieve their fitness goals.

Interactive Questions Exercise

What are some negative thoughts that might hold you back from achieving your fitness goals? How can you challenge these thoughts and replace them with more positive ones?

_____
_____
_____
_____
_____
_____
_____
_____
_____
_____
_____

What are some small changes you can make to your lifestyle that will help you reach your fitness goals?

_____
_____
_____
_____
_____
_____
_____
_____
_____

Who are some positive people in your life who can support your fitness goals? How can you surround yourself with more positive people?

_____
_____
_____
_____
_____
_____
_____
_____
_____
_____
_____

What are some affirmations that you can tell yourself to help you stay motivated?

_____
_____
_____
_____
_____
_____
_____
_____
_____
_____
_____

What are some challenges that you might face on your fitness journey? How can you overcome these challenges?

_____

_____

_____

_____

_____

_____

_____

_____

_____

_____

_____

_____

What is your ultimate fitness goal? What steps can you take today to move closer to achieving your goal?

_____

_____

_____

_____

_____

_____

_____

_____

_____

_____

_____

_____

Goals and Actionable Plan

Goal: To change your mindset from a dreamer to a doer and achieve your fitness goals.

Actionable Plan:

Identify your negative thoughts: What are the things that you tell yourself that hold you back from achieving your fitness goals? Write them down.

Challenge your negative thoughts: Why are these thoughts not true? What evidence do you have to support the opposite?

Replace your negative thoughts with positive affirmations: For each negative thought, write down a positive affirmation that you can tell yourself instead.

Surround yourself with positive people: Find people who support your fitness goals and who will encourage you to stay motivated.

Set realistic goals: Don't try to change too much too quickly. Set small, achievable goals that you can build on over time.

Make gradual changes to your lifestyle: Don't try to overhaul your entire lifestyle overnight. Make small changes that you can stick with over time.

Never give up: There will be setbacks along the way. Don't let them discourage you. Just keep moving forward and never give up on your dreams.

In addition to the actionable plan above, here are some fun and interactive ways to engage with the material in Chapter 1:

Create a vision board: Gather images and words that represent your fitness goals and create a vision board to keep you motivated.

Join a fitness challenge: There are many fitness challenges available online and in your community. Joining a challenge can help you stay accountable and motivated.

Track your progress: Keep track of your progress by keeping a journal or using a fitness tracker. This will help you see how far you've come and stay motivated to continue on your journey.

Celebrate your successes: Don't forget to celebrate your successes along the way! This will help you stay motivated and on track.

CHAPTER TWO
The Detox

Chapter 2 discusses the importance of detoxing the body before beginning the shredding phase of the program. The authors argue that toxins can build up in the body over time and can contribute to weight gain, fatigue, and other health problems. They recommend a 3-day detox to cleanse the body of toxins and prepare it for weight loss.

The authors provide a detailed plan for the detox, which includes:

Eating a clean diet: The detox diet is free of processed foods, sugar, caffeine, alcohol, and unhealthy fats. It focuses on whole, unprocessed foods that are high in nutrients.

Drinking plenty of water: Water is essential for flushing toxins out of the body. The authors recommend drinking at least 8 glasses of water per day during the detox.

Eating detoxifying foods: There are certain foods that are known to help detoxify the body. The authors recommend including these foods in your detox diet, such as:

Green vegetables: Green vegetables are high in antioxidants, which can help to protect the body from damage caused by toxins.

Fruits: Fruits are a good source of fiber, which can help to cleanse the digestive system.

Herbs and spices: Herbs and spices have detoxifying properties. Some examples include:

Ginger: Ginger can help to improve digestion and relieve nausea.

Turmeric: Turmeric has anti-inflammatory and antioxidant properties.

Cayenne pepper: Cayenne pepper can help to boost metabolism and burn fat.

The authors also recommend avoiding certain foods and beverages during the detox, such as:

Processed foods: Processed foods are often high in unhealthy fats, sugar, and sodium. They can also be high in toxins.

Sugar: Sugar can contribute to weight gain and inflammation. It can also feed the bad bacteria in your gut.

Caffeine: Caffeine can dehydrate the body and make it difficult to sleep.

Alcohol: Alcohol is high in calories and can contribute to weight gain. It can also dehydrate the body and make it difficult to sleep.

The authors conclude the chapter by saying that the detox is an important step in the shredding process. They recommend following the detox plan carefully and drinking plenty of water to ensure that you get the most out of it.

Here are some additional thoughts on Chapter 2:

The authors do a good job of explaining the importance of detoxing the body before beginning a weight loss program.

The detox plan is well-designed and easy to follow.

The authors provide helpful tips for avoiding toxins and staying hydrated during the detox.

Overall, Chapter 2 is an informative and helpful chapter that provides readers with everything they need to know about detoxing before beginning the shredding phase of the program.

Key Points of Chapter 2

The importance of detoxing: The authors argue that toxins can build up in the body over time and can contribute to weight gain, fatigue, and other health problems. They recommend a 3-day detox to cleanse the body of toxins and prepare it for weight loss.

What to eat during the detox: The detox diet is free of processed foods, sugar, caffeine, alcohol, and unhealthy fats. It focuses on whole, unprocessed foods that are high in nutrients. Some examples of detoxifying foods include green vegetables, fruits, and herbs and spices.

What to avoid during the detox: The authors recommend avoiding processed foods, sugar, caffeine, alcohol, and unhealthy fats during the detox.

The importance of drinking plenty of water: Water is essential for flushing toxins out of the body. The authors recommend drinking at least 8 glasses of water per day during the detox.

How to deal with common detox symptoms: Some common detox symptoms include fatigue, headaches, and mood swings. The authors recommend listening to your body and resting when you need to. They also recommend drinking herbal teas and taking supplements to help ease detox symptoms.

Overall, the key points of Chapter 2 are that detoxing is an important step in the shredding process, that there are certain foods and beverages that can help or hinder the detox process, and that it is important to listen to your body and rest when you need to during the detox.

Here are some additional thoughts on the key points of Chapter 2:

The authors do a good job of explaining the importance of detoxing and the different ways to detox.

The authors provide helpful tips for dealing with common detox symptoms.

The chapter is well-written and easy to follow.

Interactive Questions Exercise

What are some detoxifying foods that you enjoy eating? How can you incorporate more of these foods into your diet?

_____
_____
_____
_____
_____
_____
_____
_____
_____
_____
_____
_____
_____

Alex Willowbrooks

———————————————————————

———————————————————————

What are some common detox symptoms that you have experienced? How did you deal with them?

_____

_____

_____

_____

_____

_____

_____

_____

_____

_____

_____

What are some ways to make the detox process more enjoyable? For example, you could try cooking new recipes, listening to music, or spending time in nature.

_____

_____

_____

_____

_____

_____

_____

_____

_____

_____

_____

_____

25

What are your goals for the detox? Are you hoping to lose weight, improve your energy levels, or simply cleanse your body?

_____

_____

_____

_____

_____

_____

_____

_____

_____

_____

_____

How will you track your progress during the detox? This could involve keeping a journal, taking progress pictures, or weighing yourself regularly.

_____

_____

_____

_____

_____

_____

_____

_____

_____

_____

_____

What are some ways to celebrate your success after completing the detox? This could involve treating yourself to a healthy meal, getting a massage, or spending time with loved ones.

_____

_____

_____

_____

_____

_____

_____

_____

_____

_____

_____

Goals and Actionable Plan

Goal: To complete a 3-day detox and feel energized, clear-headed, and ready to start the shredding phase of the program.

Actionable Plan:

Set up your detox space: Find a quiet place in your home where you can relax and focus on your detox. Make sure you have all of the supplies you need, such as fruits, vegetables, herbal teas, and water.

Create a detox playlist: Make a playlist of your favorite relaxing music to listen to during your detox. This will help you to de-stress and focus on your health.

Start your detox: On the first day of your detox, focus on eating light, healthy meals and drinking plenty of water. Avoid processed foods, sugar, caffeine, alcohol, and unhealthy fats.

Take detox baths: Detox baths are a great way to cleanse your body and mind. Add essential oils to your bathwater, such as lavender, chamomile, or peppermint.

Get plenty of rest: It is important to get plenty of rest during your detox. Your body is working hard to cleanse itself, so it is important to give it the time it needs to recover.

Be patient: Detoxing can be challenging, but it is important to be patient with yourself. Don't get discouraged if you experience any detox symptoms. Just listen to your body and take things one day at a time.

Conclusion:

This is just a sample plan, and you can customize it to fit your own needs and preferences. The most important thing is to find a plan that works for you and stick with it. With a little effort, you can complete your detox and feel your best.

CHAPTER THREE
The Shredding

Chapter 3 discusses the shredding phase of the program, which is where the real weight loss happens. The authors recommend a combination of diet and exercise to help readers achieve their goals.

The authors provide a detailed plan for the shredding phase, which includes:

Diet: The shredding diet is low in calories and high in protein. It focuses on whole, unprocessed foods that are high in nutrients. Some examples of shredding diet foods include:

Lean protein: Lean protein helps to build and repair muscle tissue. Some examples of lean protein include chicken, fish, tofu, and beans.

Complex carbohydrates: Complex carbohydrates provide sustained energy. Some examples of complex carbohydrates include whole grains, fruits, and vegetables.

Healthy fats: Healthy fats help to keep you feeling full and satisfied. Some examples of healthy fats include avocados, nuts, and seeds.

Exercise: The shredding exercise plan is designed to help you build muscle and burn fat. It includes a variety of workouts, such as:

Weight lifting: Weight lifting helps to build muscle.

Cardio: Cardio helps to burn fat.

HIIT: HIIT is a type of cardio that is high-intensity and short-duration. It is a great way to burn fat and build muscle.

The authors also recommend avoiding certain foods and beverages during the shredding phase, such as:

Processed foods: Processed foods are often high in unhealthy fats, sugar, and sodium. They can also be high in calories.

Sugar: Sugar can contribute to weight gain and inflammation.

Caffeine: Caffeine can dehydrate the body and make it difficult to sleep.

Alcohol: Alcohol is high in calories and can contribute to weight gain. It can also dehydrate the body and make it difficult to sleep.

The authors conclude the chapter by saying that the shredding phase is the most important part of the program. They recommend following the diet and exercise plan carefully and being patient with yourself.

Here are some additional thoughts on Chapter 3:

The authors do a good job of explaining the importance of diet and exercise in the shredding phase.

The diet and exercise plan is well-designed and easy to follow.

The authors provide helpful tips for staying motivated during the shredding phase.

Overall, Chapter 3 is an informative and helpful chapter that provides readers with everything they need to know about the shredding phase of the program.

Here are some examples that the author included in Chapter 3:

The author provides a sample meal plan for the shredding phase.

The author provides a sample workout routine for the shredding phase.

The author provides tips for staying motivated during the shredding phase.

Key Points of Chapter 3

The importance of diet and exercise: The authors emphasize that diet and exercise are essential for achieving your shredding goals. They recommend a low-calorie, high-protein diet and a variety of workouts, such as weight lifting, cardio, and HIIT.

The importance of consistency: The authors stress that consistency is key to success in the shredding phase. They recommend following the diet and exercise plan as closely as possible and not giving up if you experience setbacks.

The importance of patience: The authors acknowledge that the shredding phase can be challenging, but they encourage readers to be patient with themselves. They remind readers that it takes time to build muscle and burn fat.

The importance of motivation: The authors provide helpful tips for staying motivated during the shredding phase, such as setting goals, tracking your progress, and finding a support system.

Overall, the key points of Chapter 3 are that diet, exercise, consistency, patience, and motivation are all essential for achieving your shredding goals.

Here are some additional thoughts on the key points of Chapter 3:

The authors do a good job of explaining the importance of each of these key points.

The authors provide helpful tips for how to implement each of these key points.

The chapter is well-written and easy to follow.

Interactive Questions Exercise

What are some of your favorite shredding diet foods? How can you incorporate more of these foods into your diet?

_____
_____
_____
_____
_____
_____
_____
_____
_____
_____
_____
_____
_____
_____
_____

_____

_____

_____

What are some of your favorite shredding exercise routines? How can you make them more fun and engaging?

_____

_____

_____

_____

_____

_____

_____

_____

_____

_____

_____

What are some challenges you have faced in the shredding phase? How have you overcome these challenges?

_____

_____

_____

_____

_____

_____

_____

_____

_____

_____

_____

_____

What are some tips you would give to someone else who is starting the shredding phase?

_____

_____

_____

_____

_____

_____

_____

_____

_____

_____

What are some of your goals for the shredding phase? How will you measure your success?

_____

_____

_____

_____

_____

_____

_____

_____

_____

_____

_____

How will you celebrate your success when you reach your goals?

_____
_____
_____
_____
_____
_____
_____
_____
_____
_____
_____
_____

Goals and Actionable Plan

Goal: To shred 10 pounds of fat in 30 days.

Actionable Plan:

Set up a shredding space: Find a quiet place in your home where you can relax and focus on your shredding goals. Make sure you have all of the supplies you need, such as weights, resistance bands, a yoga mat, and water.

Create a shredding playlist: Make a playlist of your favorite upbeat music to listen to while you work out. This will help you to stay motivated and focus on your workout.

Start your shredding journey: On the first day of your shredding journey, focus on eating a healthy breakfast and getting a good workout in. Avoid processed foods, sugar, and unhealthy fats.

Track your progress: Keep a journal or use an app to track your progress. This will help you to see how far you've come and stay motivated to continue.

Celebrate your successes: When you reach a goal, take some time to celebrate your success. This will help you to stay motivated and on track.

Additional Tips:

Find a workout buddy or join a fitness class. Having someone to work out with can help you stay motivated and accountable.

Make sure you are getting enough sleep. Sleep is essential for muscle growth and recovery.

Listen to your body and take rest days when you need them. Pushing yourself too hard can lead to injury.

Be patient and don't give up. Shredding takes time and effort, but it is definitely achievable.

CHAPTER FOUR
The Maintenance

Chapter 4 discusses the maintenance phase of the program, which is where you focus on keeping the weight off and making healthy choices a lifestyle. The authors recommend continuing to follow a healthy diet and exercise routine, but in a more relaxed and sustainable way.

The authors provide a few tips for maintaining your shredded physique:

Make healthy choices a lifestyle: Don't think of your healthy diet and exercise routine as a temporary fix. Make it a part of your everyday life.

Find a balance that works for you: There is no one-size-fits-all approach to maintenance. Find a balance between healthy eating and exercise that you can stick with long-term.

Don't be afraid to indulge: Everyone deserves a cheat meal or two every now and then. Just don't let it derail your progress.

Listen to your body: If you're feeling tired or stressed, take a break from your routine. Don't push yourself too hard.

Celebrate your successes: When you reach a goal, take some time to celebrate your success. This will help you stay motivated and on track.

The authors also include a few examples of how to maintain your shredded physique:

Continue to eat a healthy diet: This means eating plenty of fruits, vegetables, and whole grains. It also means limiting processed foods, sugar, and unhealthy fats.

Continue to exercise regularly: Aim for at least 30 minutes of moderate-intensity exercise most days of the week. You can also break up your exercise into shorter sessions throughout the day.

Find a support system: Having friends or family members who are also on a healthy journey can help you stay motivated.

Don't be afraid to ask for help: If you're struggling to maintain your shredded physique, don't be afraid to ask for help from a qualified professional.

Key Points of Chapter 4

Make healthy choices a lifestyle: This means making healthy eating and exercise a part of your everyday life. It doesn't mean you have to be perfect all the time, but it does mean making healthy choices most of the time.

Find a balance that works for you: There is no one-size-fits-all approach to maintenance. Find a balance between healthy eating and exercise that you can stick with long-term. This may mean eating a little more or exercising a little less than you did during the shredding phase.

Don't be afraid to indulge: Everyone deserves a cheat meal or two every now and then. Just don't let it derail your progress. If you do indulge, make sure to get back on track the next day.

Listen to your body: If you're feeling tired or stressed, take a break from your routine. Don't push yourself too hard.

Celebrate your successes: When you reach a goal, take some time to celebrate your success. This will help you stay motivated and on track.

Overall, the key points of Chapter 4 are that making healthy choices a lifestyle, finding a balance that works for you, indulging occasionally, listening to your body, and celebrating your successes are all important for maintaining your shredded physique for the long term.

Here are some additional thoughts on the key points of Chapter 4:

The authors do a good job of explaining the importance of each of these key points.

The authors provide helpful tips for how to implement each of these key points.

The chapter is well-written and easy to follow.

Interactive Questions Exercise

What are some healthy foods that you enjoy eating that you could incorporate into your maintenance diet?

_____
_____
_____
_____
_____
_____
_____
_____
_____
_____
_____

What are some fun and engaging ways that you could exercise regularly during the maintenance phase?

_____
_____
_____
_____
_____
_____
_____
_____
_____
_____
_____
_____
_____

What are some challenges that you might face in maintaining your shredded physique? How would you overcome these challenges?

_____
_____
_____
_____
_____
_____
_____
_____
_____
_____
_____
_____

What are some tips that you would give to someone else who is starting the maintenance phase?

_____
_____
_____
_____
_____
_____
_____
_____
_____
_____
_____
_____

What are some of your goals for the maintenance phase?
How will you measure your success?

_____

_____

_____

_____

_____

_____

_____

_____

_____

_____

_____

_____

How will you celebrate your success when you reach your goals?

_____

_____

_____

_____

_____

_____

_____

_____

_____

_____

_____

_____

Here are some additional prompts that you can use to engage with the material in Chapter 4:

Create a vision board for your shredded physique. What does your dream body look like? What does it feel like to have a shredded physique?

Write a letter to your future self. In the letter, describe how you are going to maintain your shredded physique for the long term.

Create a healthy meal plan for the week. Make sure to include a variety of healthy foods that you enjoy eating.

Design a workout routine that you can stick with long-term. Make sure to include a variety of exercises that work all of your muscle groups.

Find a support system to help you stay motivated. This could include friends, family, or a fitness community.

Don't be afraid to ask for help. If you're struggling to maintain your shredded physique, don't be afraid to ask for help from a qualified professional.

Goals and Actionable Plan

Goal: To maintain my shredded physique for the next 12 months.

Actionable Plan:

Create a vision board: This will help me to stay focused on my goal and motivated to make healthy choices.

Set monthly goals: This will help me to track my progress and make sure I am on track.

Find a support system: This could include friends, family, or a fitness community.

Make healthy choices a lifestyle: This means making healthy eating and exercise a part of my everyday life.

Don't be afraid to indulge: Everyone deserves a cheat meal or two every now and then. Just don't let it derail your progress.

Listen to my body: If I'm feeling tired or stressed, take a break from my routine. Don't push myself too hard.

Celebrate my successes: When I reach a goal, take some time to celebrate my success. This will help me stay motivated and on track.

Additional Tips:

Make it fun: Find ways to make healthy eating and exercise enjoyable. This could include cooking new recipes, trying new activities, or working out with friends.

Be patient: It takes time to maintain a shredded physique. Don't get discouraged if you have setbacks. Just keep working towards your goal.

Don't give up: Maintaining your shredded physique is a challenge, but it is definitely possible. Just stay focused, make healthy choices, and don't give up.

CHAPTER FIVE
Recipes

Chapter 5 provides readers with a variety of healthy recipes that they can incorporate into their diet. The recipes are all designed to be low in calories and high in protein, making them perfect for the shredding phase of the program.

The author includes a few tips for making the recipes:

Use fresh ingredients whenever possible. This will ensure that your recipes taste their best.

Don't be afraid to experiment. There are endless possibilities when it comes to healthy cooking.

Have fun with it! Cooking should be enjoyable. If you're not having fun, you're less likely to stick with it.

The author also includes a few examples of recipes:

Chicken Breast with Roasted Vegetables: This recipe is a great source of protein and fiber. The roasted vegetables add flavor and nutrients.

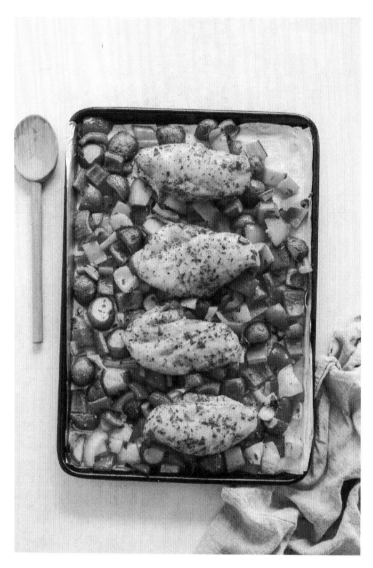

Chicken Breast with Roasted Vegetables

Salmon with Brown Rice and Asparagus: This recipe is another great source of protein and fiber. The salmon is rich in omega-3 fatty acids, which are beneficial for heart health.

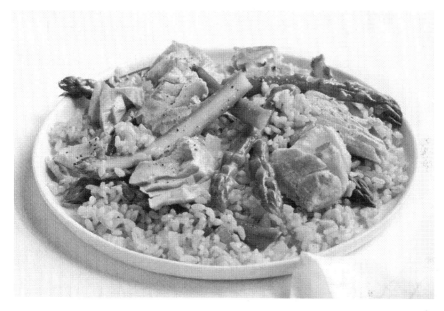

Salmon with Brown Rice and Asparagus

Lentil Soup: This soup is a great way to get your daily dose of protein and fiber. It's also a good source of iron.

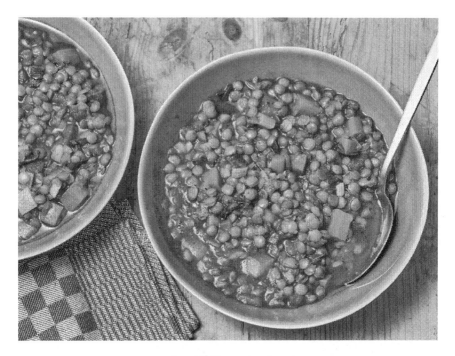

Lentil Soup recipe

Smoothies: Smoothies are a great way to get a quick and easy meal or snack. They're also a great way to incorporate fruits, vegetables, and protein into your diet.

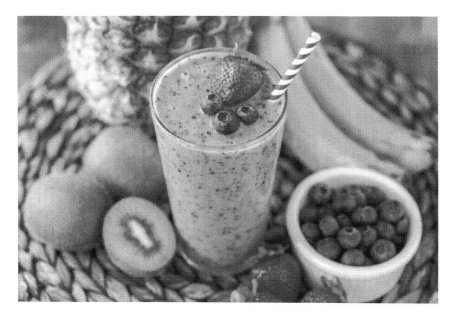

Smoothies' recipe

Overall, Chapter 5 provides readers with a variety of healthy and delicious recipes that they can incorporate into their diet. The recipes are all designed to be low in calories and high in protein, making them perfect for the shredding phase of the program.

Key Points of Chapter 5

The recipes are all low in calories and high in protein. This makes them perfect for the shredding phase of the program.

The recipes are all easy to make. This means that you can make them even if you're short on time or don't have a lot of cooking experience.

The recipes are all delicious. This means that you'll actually enjoy eating them, which will make it more likely that you'll stick to the program.

Here are some additional thoughts on the key points of Chapter 5:

The author does a good job of providing recipes that are both healthy and delicious.

The recipes are all well-written and easy to follow.

The author includes helpful tips for making the recipes.

Interactive Questions Exercise

What is your favorite recipe from Chapter 5? Why do you like it so much?

_____

_____

_____

_____

_____

_____

_____

_____

_____

_____

_____

_____

_____

_____

_____

_____

_____

_____

What recipe from Chapter 5 would you like to try? What do you think you would like about it?

_____

_____

_____

_____

_____

_____

_____

_____

_____

_____

_____

How could you make one of the recipes from Chapter 5 more personalized? What ingredients would you add or subtract?

_____

_____

_____

_____

_____

_____

_____

_____

_____

_____

_____

What are some other healthy and delicious recipes that you would like to share?

_____
_____
_____
_____
_____
_____
_____
_____
_____
_____
_____
_____

What are some tips for making the recipes in Chapter 5 more fun and engaging?

_____
_____
_____
_____
_____
_____
_____
_____
_____
_____
_____
_____

Here are some additional prompts that you can use to engage with the material in Chapter 5:

Create a recipe binder: Collect all of your favorite recipes from Chapter 5 and other sources. This will make it easy to find recipes when you're looking for something to cook.

Start a cooking blog: Share your recipes with others by starting a cooking blog. This is a great way to connect with other people who are interested in healthy cooking.

Host a cooking party: Invite friends over to cook and eat together. This is a fun way to share your love of healthy cooking with others.

Volunteer your cooking skills: Volunteer to cook for a local soup kitchen or food bank. This is a great way to give back to your community and share your love of healthy cooking with others.

Goals and Actionable Plan

Goal: To cook at least one recipe from Chapter 5 each week for the next month.

Actionable Plan:

Choose a recipe: Browse through Chapter 5 and choose a recipe that you are interested in trying.

Gather your ingredients: Make sure you have all of the ingredients you need to make your recipe.

Cook your recipe: Follow the instructions in the recipe carefully.

Enjoy your meal: Sit down and enjoy your delicious and healthy meal.

Reflect on your experience: Think about how you enjoyed the recipe and what you could do to make it even better next time.

Additional Tips:

Get creative: Don't be afraid to experiment with different ingredients and flavors.

Have fun: Cooking should be enjoyable. If you're not having fun, you're less likely to stick with it.

Share your meals: Invite friends and family over to try your new recipes.

Track your progress: Keep a journal of the recipes you try and how you enjoyed them. This will help you to stay motivated and on track.

CHAPTER SIX

Workouts

Chapter 6 provides readers with a variety of workouts that they can incorporate into their fitness routine. The workouts are all designed to be high-intensity and low-rep, making them perfect for the shredding phase of the program.

The author includes a few tips for getting the most out of the workouts:

Warm up: Before you start any workout, it's important to warm up your body. This will help to prevent injuries.

Focus on form: When you're lifting weights, it's important to focus on form over weight. This will help you to avoid injuries and get the most out of your workout.

Listen to your body: If you're feeling pain, stop the workout and take a break. Don't push yourself too hard.

Stay hydrated: It's important to stay hydrated throughout your workout. Drink plenty of water before, during, and after your workout.

The author also includes a few examples of workouts:

Chest and Triceps: This workout focuses on building chest and triceps muscle.

Back and Biceps: This workout focuses on building back and biceps muscle.

Legs and Shoulders: This workout focuses on building legs and shoulders muscle.

Overall, Chapter 6 provides readers with a variety of high-intensity workouts that they can incorporate into their fitness routine. The workouts are all designed to help readers shred fat and build muscle.

Here are some additional thoughts on the key points of Chapter 6:

The author does a good job of explaining the importance of warming up, focusing on form, listening to your body, and staying hydrated.

The workouts are all well-explained and easy to follow.

The author includes helpful tips for getting the most out of the workouts.

Overall, Chapter 6 is a valuable resource for readers who are looking for high-intensity workouts to help them shred fat and build muscle.

Here are some additional tips for getting the most out of the workouts:

Find a workout buddy: Working out with a buddy can help you stay motivated and accountable.

Set realistic goals: Don't try to do too much too soon. Start with a few workouts per week and gradually increase the number of workouts as you get stronger.

Don't give up: Getting in shape takes time and effort. Don't give up if you don't see results immediately. Just keep working hard and you will eventually reach your goals.

Key Points of Chapter 6

The workouts are all high-intensity and low-rep. This means that they are designed to get your heart rate up and burn fat quickly.

The workouts are all compound exercises. This means that they work multiple muscle groups at the same time.

The workouts are all full-body workouts. This means that they work all of the major muscle groups in your body.

The workouts are designed to be progressive. This means that they get more challenging as you get stronger.

The workouts are designed to be sustainable. This means that you can do them consistently without getting injured or burned out.

Here are some additional thoughts on the key points of Chapter 6:

The author does a good job of explaining the benefits of high-intensity, low-rep workouts.

The author includes a variety of compound exercises in the workouts, which is important for building muscle and burning fat.

The author includes full-body workouts in the program, which is important for overall fitness.

The author's progressive workout plan ensures that you will continue to see results as you get stronger.

The author's sustainable workout plan makes it easy to stick with the program long-term.

Overall, Chapter 6 provides readers with a comprehensive workout program that is designed to help them shred fat and build muscle. The workouts are all high-intensity, low-rep, compound exercises that are full-body and progressive. The program is also sustainable, making it easy to stick with long-term.

Here are some additional tips for getting the most out of the workouts:

Warm up: Before you start any workout, it's important to warm up your body. This will help to prevent injuries.

Focus on form: When you're lifting weights, it's important to focus on form over weight. This will help you to avoid injuries and get the most out of your workout.

Listen to your body: If you're feeling pain, stop the workout and take a break. Don't push yourself too hard.

Stay hydrated: It's important to stay hydrated throughout your workout. Drink plenty of water before, during, and after your workout.

Get enough rest: Your body needs time to recover from your workouts. Make sure you're getting 7-8 hours of sleep per night.

Eat a healthy diet: A healthy diet will help you to fuel your workouts and recover from them. Make sure you're eating plenty of fruits, vegetables, and whole grains.

Interactive Questions Exercise

Alex Willowbrooks

What is your favorite workout from Chapter 6? Why do you like it so much?

_____
_____
_____
_____
_____
_____
_____
_____
_____
_____
_____

What workout from Chapter 6 would you like to try? What do you think you would like about it?

_____
_____
_____
_____
_____
_____
_____
_____
_____
_____
_____

How could you make one of the workouts from Chapter 6 more personalized? What exercises would you add or subtract?

_____

_____

_____

_____

_____

_____

_____

_____

_____

_____

_____

What are some other high-intensity workouts that you would like to share?

_____

_____

_____

_____

_____

_____

_____

_____

_____

_____

_____

What are some tips for making the workouts in Chapter 6 more fun and engaging?

_____
_____
_____
_____
_____
_____
_____
_____
_____
_____
_____
_____

Here are some additional prompts that you can use to engage with the material in Chapter 6:

Create a workout playlist: Make a playlist of your favorite high-energy music to listen to during your workouts.

Find a workout buddy: Working out with a friend can help you stay motivated and accountable.

Set realistic goals: Don't try to do too much too soon. Start with a few workouts per week and gradually increase the number of workouts as you get stronger.

Don't give up: Getting in shape takes time and effort. Don't give up if you don't see results immediately. Just keep working hard and you will eventually reach your goals.

Take progress pictures: Taking progress pictures can help you to see how far you've come and stay motivated.

Track your workouts: Keeping track of your workouts can help you to see how you're doing and make adjustments to your routine as needed.

Reward yourself: When you reach a goal, reward yourself with something you enjoy. This will help you to stay motivated.

Goals and Actionable Plan

Goal: To complete a full-body workout at least 3 times per week for the next month.

Actionable Plan:

Choose a workout: Browse through Chapter 6 and choose a workout that you are interested in trying.

Gather your equipment: Make sure you have all of the equipment you need for your workout.

Find a workout space: Find a space where you can workout safely and comfortably.

Warm up: Before you start your workout, warm up your body by doing some light cardio and dynamic stretches.

Complete the workout: Follow the instructions for your workout carefully.

Cool down: After you finish your workout, cool down your body by doing some light cardio and static stretches.

Track your progress: Keep track of your workouts so you can see how you're doing and make adjustments to your routine as needed.

Additional Tips:

Find a workout buddy: Working out with a friend can help you stay motivated and accountable.

Set realistic goals: Don't try to do too much too soon. Start with a few workouts per week and gradually increase the number of workouts as you get stronger.

Don't give up: Getting in shape takes time and effort. Don't give up if you don't see results immediately. Just keep working hard and you will eventually reach your goals.

Make it fun: Choose workouts that you enjoy and that challenge you. This will help you to stay motivated and on track.

Celebrate your successes: When you reach a goal, celebrate your success! This will help you to stay motivated and on track.

CHAPTER SEVEN
Supplements

Chapter 7 provides readers with information on a variety of supplements that can be used to help with weight loss and muscle building. The author discusses the benefits of each supplement, as well as potential side effects and risks.

The author includes a few examples of supplements:

Protein powder: Protein powder can help you to build muscle and recover from workouts.

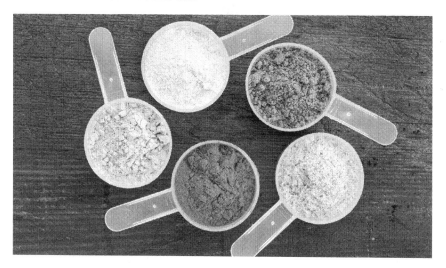

Protein powder supplement

Creatine: Creatine can help you to increase your strength and power.

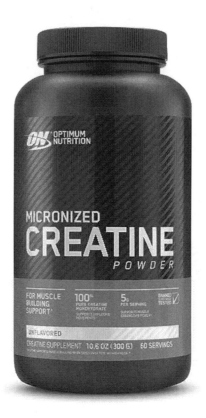

Creatine supplement

BCAAs: BCAAs can help you to prevent muscle breakdown and improve your recovery.

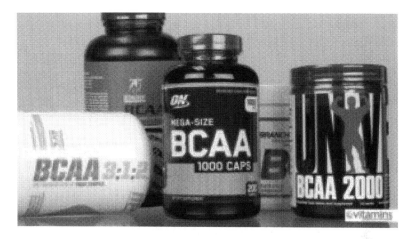

BCAAs supplement

Fish oil: Fish oil can help you to reduce inflammation and improve your overall health.

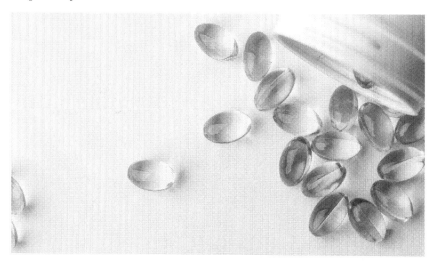

Fish oil supplement

Multivitamin: A multivitamin can help to ensure that you are getting all of the nutrients you need.

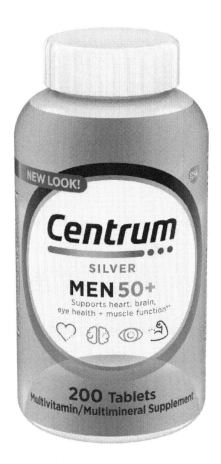

Multivitamin supplement

The author also includes a few tips for choosing supplements:

Do your research: Make sure you do your research on any supplement before you take it.

Talk to your doctor: Talk to your doctor before taking any supplements, especially if you have any health conditions.

Start slowly: Start with a low dose of any supplement and increase the dose gradually as needed.

Listen to your body: If you experience any side effects, stop taking the supplement and talk to your doctor.

Overall, Chapter 7 provides readers with a comprehensive overview of supplements that can be used to help with weight loss and muscle building. The author does a good job of discussing the benefits and risks of each supplement, as well as providing tips for choosing supplements safely.

Here are some additional thoughts on the key points of Chapter 7:

Supplements should not be used as a substitute for a healthy diet and exercise.

Supplements should be taken under the guidance of a doctor or registered dietitian.

Supplements can interact with medications, so it is important to talk to your doctor before taking any supplements.

Supplements can be expensive, so it is important to do your research and find supplements that are safe and effective.

Key Points of Chapter 7

Supplements can be a helpful addition to a healthy diet and exercise routine, but they should not be used as a substitute for either.

There are many different types of supplements available, and each one has its own benefits and risks.

It is important to do your research and talk to your doctor before taking any supplements, especially if you have any health conditions.

Some common supplements that can be helpful for weight loss and muscle building include protein powder, creatine, BCAAs, fish oil, and multivitamins.

It is important to start with a low dose of any supplement and increase the dose gradually as needed.

If you experience any side effects while taking a supplement, stop taking it and talk to your doctor.

Here are some additional thoughts on the key points of Chapter 7:

Supplements can be a helpful way to boost your nutrient intake and reach your fitness goals.

However, it is important to remember that supplements are not a magic bullet.

They will not work if you are not following a healthy diet and exercise routine.

It is also important to be aware of the potential side effects of any supplement before you take it.

If you are considering taking supplements, I recommend doing your research and talking to your doctor to make sure they are right for you.

Interactive Questions Exercise

What is your favorite supplement and why?

_____
_____
_____
_____
_____
_____
_____
_____
_____
_____
_____

What supplement would you like to try?

_____
_____
_____
_____
_____
_____
_____
_____
_____
_____
_____

What are some of the benefits and risks of taking supplements?

_____

_____

_____

_____

_____

_____

_____

_____

_____

_____

_____

What are some tips for choosing supplements safely?

_____

_____

_____

_____

_____

_____

_____

_____

_____

_____

_____

_____

Alex Willowbrooks

What are some of the most common supplements that people take for weight loss and muscle building?

_____
_____
_____
_____
_____
_____
_____
_____
_____
_____
_____

What are some of the best ways to get the nutrients you need without taking supplements?

_____
_____
_____
_____
_____
_____
_____
_____
_____
_____
_____

Here are some additional prompts that you can use to engage with the material in Chapter 7:

Create a supplement journal: Keep track of the supplements you take, how much you take, and how you feel. This will help you to see if the supplements are working for you and to make sure you are not taking too much of any one supplement.

Talk to your doctor about supplements: Talk to your doctor about the supplements you are taking and any potential side effects. This will help you to stay safe and healthy.

Do your research: Do your research on any supplement before you take it. This will help you to make sure that the supplement is safe and effective for you.

Start slowly: Start with a low dose of any supplement and increase the dose gradually as needed. This will help you to avoid any side effects.

Listen to your body: If you experience any side effects while taking a supplement, stop taking it and talk to your doctor.

Goals and Actionable Plan

Goal: To learn more about supplements and to make informed decisions about whether or not to take them.

Actionable Plan:

Read Chapter 7: Supplements in the book "30 Days 2 Shredz". This will give you a comprehensive overview of supplements and their potential benefits and risks.

Do your own research on supplements. There are many resources available online and in libraries that can help you to learn more about supplements.

Talk to your doctor about supplements. Your doctor can help you to assess your individual needs and make recommendations about which supplements, if any, are right for you.

Start slowly. If you decide to take supplements, start with a low dose and increase the dose gradually as needed. This will help you to avoid any side effects.

Listen to your body. If you experience any side effects while taking a supplement, stop taking it and talk to your doctor.

Additional Tips:

Be skeptical of marketing claims. Not all supplements are created equal. Do your research and be wary of supplements that make exaggerated claims about their benefits.

Buy supplements from reputable sources. There are many counterfeit supplements on the market. Make sure to buy your supplements from a reputable source that you trust.

Store your supplements properly. Supplements should be stored in a cool, dry place.

Do not take expired supplements. Supplements can lose their potency over time. Do not take expired supplements.

CHAPTER EIGHT
Common Questions

Chapter 8 provides readers with answers to some of the most common questions they may have about the program. The author addresses questions about diet, exercise, supplements, and more.

Here are some of the questions that the author addresses in Chapter 8:

What is the best way to lose weight?

How much protein should I eat?

What are the best exercises for weight loss?

What supplements can help me lose weight?

How do I stay motivated?

What should I do if I plateau?

How can I prevent weight gain in the future?

The author provides clear and concise answers to all of these questions. The author also includes helpful tips and advice that can help readers reach their weight loss goals.

Here are some examples of the questions that the author includes in Chapter 8:

Q: What is the best way to lose weight?

A: There is no one-size-fits-all answer to this question. The best way to lose weight will vary depending on your individual needs and goals. However, some general tips include eating a healthy diet, exercising regularly, and getting enough sleep.

Q: How much protein should I eat?

A: The amount of protein you need to eat will vary depending on your age, sex, activity level, and individual goals. However, as a general rule of thumb, most people should aim to consume 0.8 grams of protein per kilogram of body weight per day.

Q: What are the best exercises for weight loss?

A: There are many different exercises that can help you lose weight. Some of the best exercises for weight loss include cardio exercises, strength-training exercises, and high-intensity interval training (HIIT).

Q: What supplements can help me lose weight?

A: There are a number of supplements that can help you lose weight. Some of the most popular supplements for weight loss include protein powder, creatine, and BCAAs. However, it is important to note that supplements should not be used as a substitute for a healthy diet and exercise.

Q: How do I stay motivated?

A: Staying motivated can be challenging, but it is important to find ways to stay on track. Some tips for staying motivated include setting realistic goals, tracking your progress, and finding an accountability partner.

Q: What should I do if I plateau?

A: If you reach a plateau in your weight loss, it is important to make adjustments to your diet and exercise routine. Some tips for breaking a plateau include increasing the intensity of your workouts, changing up your workout routine, and reducing your calorie intake.

Q: How can I prevent weight gain in the future?

A: There are a number of things you can do to prevent weight gain in the future. Some tips include maintaining a healthy weight, eating a healthy diet, exercising regularly, and getting enough sleep.

Overall, Chapter 8 provides readers with a comprehensive resource for answering some of the most common questions they may have about the 30 Days 2 Shredz program. The author provides clear and concise answers to all of the questions, as well as helpful tips and advice that can help readers reach their weight loss goals.

Key Points of Chapter 8

There is no one-size-fits-all answer to the question of how to lose weight. The best way to lose weight will vary depending on your individual needs and goals.

Eating a healthy diet, exercising regularly, and getting enough sleep are all important for weight loss.

The amount of protein you need to eat will vary depending on your age, sex, activity level, and individual goals. As a general rule of thumb, most people should aim to consume 0.8 grams of protein per kilogram of body weight per day.

There are many different exercises that can help you lose weight. Some of the best exercises for weight loss include cardio exercises, strength-training exercises, and high-intensity interval training (HIIT).

Supplements can help you lose weight, but they should not be used as a substitute for a healthy diet and exercise.

Staying motivated can be challenging, but it is important to find ways to stay on track. Some tips for staying motivated include setting realistic goals, tracking your progress, and finding an accountability partner.

If you reach a plateau in your weight loss, it is important to make adjustments to your diet and exercise routine. Some tips for breaking a plateau include increasing the intensity of your workouts, changing up your workout routine, and reducing your calorie intake.

There are a number of things you can do to prevent weight gain in the future. Some tips include maintaining a healthy weight, eating a healthy diet, exercising regularly, and getting enough sleep.

Here are some additional thoughts on the key points of Chapter 8:

It is important to be patient and persistent when trying to lose weight. Weight loss takes time and effort.

It is important to listen to your body and find a weight loss plan that works for you. There is no one-size-fits-all approach to weight loss.

There are many resources available to help you lose weight and keep it off. Talk to your doctor, a registered dietitian, or a certified personal trainer for more information and support.

I hope this discussion helps you to understand the key points of Chapter 8: Common Questions of the book "30 Days 2 Shredz".

Interactive Questions Exercise

What is your favorite question from Chapter 8 and why?

_____

_____

_____

_____

_____

_____

_____

_____

_____

_____

_____

What question do you have about weight loss that you would like to ask the author?

_____

_____

_____

_____

_____

_____

_____

_____

_____

_____

_____

_____

_____

_____

What is your biggest challenge when it comes to losing weight?

_____
_____
_____
_____
_____
_____
_____
_____
_____
_____
_____

What is your favorite tip for staying motivated?

_____
_____
_____
_____
_____
_____
_____
_____
_____
_____
_____
_____
_____
_____
_____
_____

Alex Willowbrooks

What is your favorite exercise for weight loss?

_____
_____
_____
_____
_____
_____
_____
_____
_____
_____

What is your favorite healthy food for weight loss?

_____
_____
_____
_____
_____
_____
_____
_____
_____
_____
_____
_____
_____
_____

Here are some additional prompts that you can use to engage with the material in Chapter 8:

Create a weight loss journal: Keep track of your weight loss progress, what you eat, and how much exercise you get. This will help you to stay motivated and see your progress.

Find an accountability partner: Find a friend or family member who is also trying to lose weight. You can support each other and hold each other accountable.

Join a weight loss support group: There are many weight loss support groups available online and in person. These groups can provide you with motivation and support.

Reward yourself for your progress: When you reach a weight loss goal, reward yourself with something you enjoy. This will help you to stay motivated.

Don't give up: Weight loss is a journey, not a destination. There will be ups and downs, but don't give up on your goals.

Goals and Actionable Plan

Goal: To learn more about weight loss and to develop a personalized weight loss plan.

Actionable Plan:

Read Chapter 8: Common Questions in the book "30 Days 2 Shredz". This will give you a comprehensive overview of common questions about weight loss and their answers.

Reflect on your own weight loss journey. What are your biggest challenges? What are your goals?

Create a personalized weight loss plan. This plan should be based on your individual needs and goals.

Track your progress. This will help you to stay motivated and see your progress.

Find an accountability partner. This could be a friend, family member, or weight loss coach.

Reward yourself for your progress. This will help you to stay motivated.

Don't give up! Weight loss is a journey, not a destination. There will be ups and downs, but don't give up on your goals.

Here are some additional tips for making your weight loss journey more fun and interactive:

Set realistic goals. Don't try to lose too much weight too quickly. Aim for a healthy and sustainable rate of weight loss.

Find activities that you enjoy. Exercise doesn't have to be boring! Find activities that you enjoy and that challenge you.

Make changes to your diet that you can stick with. Don't try to make too many changes at once. Make small changes that you can gradually incorporate into your lifestyle.

Celebrate your successes. When you reach a goal, take some time to celebrate your success. This will help you to stay motivated.

Don't be afraid to ask for help. If you're struggling, don't be afraid to ask for help from a friend, family member, or weight loss professional.

CHAPTER NINE
Conclusion

Chapter 9 provides readers with a summary of the key points of the book and offers some final thoughts on weight loss and healthy living. The author emphasizes the importance of making lasting changes to your lifestyle and not just following a fad diet.

Here are some of the key points that the author makes in Chapter 9:

Weight loss is a journey, not a destination. It takes time and effort to make lasting changes to your lifestyle.

There is no one-size-fits-all approach to weight loss. What works for one person may not work for another.

It is important to find a weight loss plan that you can stick with. If you make too many changes too quickly, you are more likely to give up.

It is important to be patient and persistent. Weight loss takes time and effort.

It is important to celebrate your successes. When you reach a goal, take some time to celebrate your success. This will help you to stay motivated.

It is important to have a support system. Having friends or family members who are supportive of your weight loss goals can make a big difference.

It is important to remember that you are not alone. Millions of people are struggling with weight loss. There are resources available to help you.

The author also includes a few examples of people who have successfully lost weight and kept it off. These examples can be inspiring to readers who are struggling to reach their own weight loss goals.

Overall, Chapter 9 provides readers with a positive and motivating message about weight loss. The author emphasizes the importance of making lasting changes to your lifestyle and not just following a fad diet. The author also includes some helpful tips for staying motivated and on track.

Here are some additional thoughts on the key points of Chapter 9:

It is important to remember that weight loss is not always linear. There will be ups and downs along the way. Don't let this discourage you. Just keep moving forward.

It is important to focus on your overall health and well-being, not just your weight. When you make healthy choices, you will feel better both physically and mentally.

It is important to enjoy the journey. Weight loss can be a challenge, but it should also be enjoyable. Find activities that you enjoy and that help you to reach your goals.

I hope this discussion helps you to understand the key points of Chapter 9: Conclusion of the book "30 Days 2 Shredz".

Alex Willowbrooks